HEALTH CARE CAREERS IN 2 YEARS ™

JUMP-STARTING A CAREER IN

VETERINARY MEDICINE

JERI FREEDMAN

D1525331

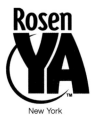

Rosen
YA™

New York

Published in 2019 by The Rosen Publishing Group, Inc.
29 East 21st Street, New York, NY 10010

Library of Congress Cataloging-in-Publication Data

Names: Freedman, Jeri, author.
Title: Jump-starting a career in veterinary medicine / Jeri Freedman.
Description: First edition. | New York: Rosen YA, 2019. | Series: Health care careers in 2 years | Audience: Grade 7–12. | Includes bibliographical references and index.
Identifiers: LCCN 2018011828| ISBN 9781508185147 (library bound) | ISBN 9781508185130 (paperback)
Subjects: LCSH: Veterinary medicine—Vocational guidance.
Classification: LCC SF756.28 .F74 2019 | DDC 636.089023—dc23
LC record available at https://lccn.loc.gov/2018011828

Manufactured in the United States of America

CONTENTS

INTRODUCTION

As she recounts on the Moncton Animal Hospital website, Jessica Moran began the hands-on training part of her veterinary technician program by working at the hospital. In the morning, she assisted with surgeries under the supervision of one of the veterinarians or technicians. Moran cleaned the surgery area and collected the equipment that would be needed for surgery. Her most memorable activity was helping with an emergency cesarean section (C-section) on a dog that was having trouble giving birth. A C-section is surgery to remove a baby from the womb if the mother cannot deliver it through the birth canal. Moran restrained the mother dog so it could be anesthetized, and she got together all the equipment that would be needed to keep her comfortable and warm. When everything was ready, she waited to receive the puppies and if necessary to try to get them breathing. Moran was delighted to help deliver five healthy little puppies.

Many students are interested in working with animals, but they believe that a career in veterinary medicine requires extensive education, which is expensive and therefore out of their reach. There are entry-level jobs in the field, however, that require two years or less of education to get started, and these jobs can be the first step on an excellent career path.

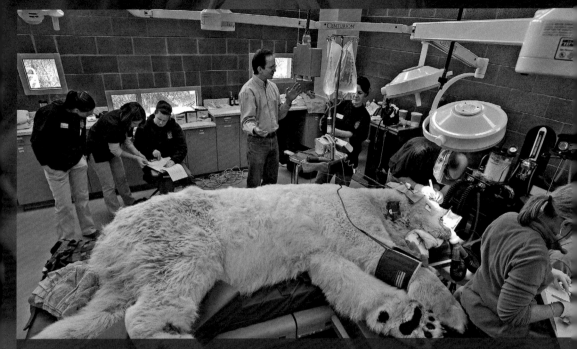

Veterinary staff at a zoo give a physical exam to a sedated polar bear. In the veterinary field one can work with exotic as well as domestic animals.

Working in the veterinary field involves more than just handling animals. The jobs in the field requiring two years or less of training range from veterinary receptionists and assistants to veterinary technicians. Those who start in such jobs can advance to supervisory or managerial positions, or acquire additional experience or training and move to related animal jobs such as animal health inspector.

Some animals will need only a routine exam or shots, but many will be injured or ill, which can be upsetting to see. Nonetheless, the veterinary field provides the opportunity to make a difference in the lives of creatures who cannot help themselves. It feels good to help a sick or injured animal get better or to ease its suffering.

Veterinary offices that treat pets such as dogs and cats are not the only places where veterinarians and their assistants and technicians work. The veterinary field also includes large animal practices, which treat farm and ranch animals such as sheep, cows, and horses; mixed animal practices, which treat both small and large animals; zoo and aquarium practices, which care for exotic animals; and animal sanctuaries and preserves for wild animals, as well as other venues. Given the large number of geographic locations and types of facilities in the field, there is a steady demand for employees, which provides job security. The veterinary field offers the opportunity to work in the practitioner's choice of indoor and outdoor environments with the types of animals he or she prefers.

The material covered here will describe the specific jobs available, the training and certification required, and practical ways to successfully locate and apply for a job that requires two years or fewer of training.

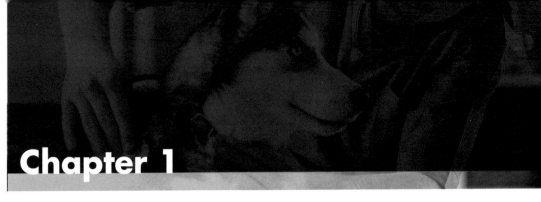

Chapter 1

TAKING CARE OF ANIMALS

I n good times and bad, people take care of their animals, on farms and ranches; in public facilities such as zoos, aquariums, and preserves; in shelters; and above all in their homes. Therefore, a position in the veterinary field can provide job security, as well as the fulfillment of making animals' lives better and longer. There are veterinary jobs that do not require advanced degrees from prestigious and expensive universities. Moreover, veterinary jobs are available in a wide variety of settings, providing the opportunity to work with the type of animals one prefers, in a facility and location of one's choice. Veterinary staff can work in large, small, or mixed animal practices; in urban or rural locations; at zoos, aquariums, or theme parks; or in wild animal preserves and sanctuaries. These jobs are available to high school graduates with some additional training, short certification courses, or two-year college programs. Such entry-level jobs can be the first step to a more advanced position in the veterinary field, through promotion or by obtaining

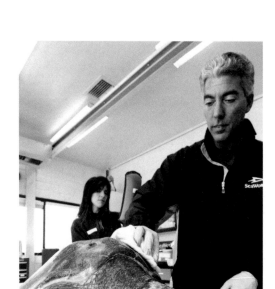

At Sea World San Diego, a veterinary technician assists in treating a sea turtle that had eaten plastic trash in the ocean, helping to save an endangered animal.

more education and training. Thus, the veterinary field can provide a secure job with benefits, which also has a solid career path and provides the satisfaction of working with animals.

Veterinary Medicine Today

The number of pets is vast and growing. The American Pet Products Association (APPA) states that in 2015 and 2016 there were 78 million dogs and 85.8 million cats kept as pets in the United States. About one-third of American homes have a cat, and about 44 percent have a dog. According to the American Society for the Prevention of Cruelty to Animals (ASPCA), about 6.5 million dogs and cats enter animal shelters across the United States each year. About 720,000, mostly dogs, are returned to their owners, and another 3.2 million (dogs and cats equally) are adopted.

The large number of pets is not the only driving force in the veterinary field. In the past few decades, researchers have made the public aware of the negative effect that human beings are having on the environment in which animals live and the resulting decrease in the numbers of many species in the wild. This circumstance has created an interest in protecting and breeding many wild species so that they do not become extinct. There has been a steady growth in the creation of preserves for animals, and many foundations, zoos, and related institutions have started animal protection and breeding programs. During the same period, there has been a growth in the concern over the way domestic farm animals are treated. The inspection of facilities in which such animals are bred, raised, and housed has increased. These factors provide an

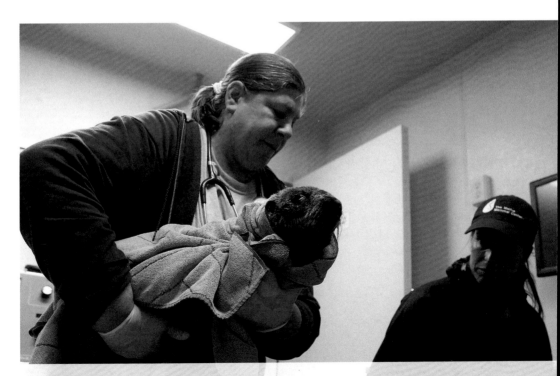

A veterinarian technician holds a malnourished northern fur seal pup during a medical evaluation at the Marine Mammal Center, which rescues and treats sea animals.

opportunity for students who want to work in the veterinary field in positions that don't require a four-year degree.

The Outlook for Veterinary Jobs

The US Bureau of Labor Statistics (BLS), in a January 30, 2018, report, projected that the number of veterinary assistants and laboratory animal caretakers employed will grow 19 percent from 2016 to 2026, much faster than the average for all occupations. In addition, high turnover in these jobs should result in good job opportunities. In its October 24, 2017, report, the BLS predicted that the number of veterinary technologist and technician positions will grow 20 percent from 2016 to 2026. Thus, employment in the veterinary field will grow significantly faster than the average for all occupations. The BLS expected the number of households with pets and the amount of money people spend on pets to continue to rise as well.

The BLS, as per its January 2018 report, expected employment of environmental science and protection technicians to grow 12 percent from 2016 to 2026, which is also faster than the average for all occupations, so the job prospects for environmental science and protection technicians are good, too. Therefore, there will continue to be healthy demand for veterinary support staff to assist with the care of animals in areas such as state and national parks and preserves.

Types of Veterinary Practices

There are many different types of veterinary practices. Small animal practices are the primary type of practice

A DAY IN THE LIFE OF AN ANIMAL CARE ATTENDANT

José's day starts with the preparation of the food for the animals who spent the night in the facility. He then cleans their cages. As he feeds the animals and cleans their cages, he observes them to see if they have any conditions that need to be reported to the veterinarians. Because the veterinary practice at which he works also boards animals, he walks and exercises the dogs. Even though the practice is not open on Sunday, José or another animal attendant works on weekends, feeding and exercising the animals staying at the facility, and cleaning their cages. A dog with several puppies is brought in by a local animal rescue group for which the practice provides services. They were found in an abandoned warehouse where the mother had taken refuge. The vet examines them and declares that the puppies' mother has done a good job and the puppies are healthy but have fleas. José gives them flea baths. As new animals are admitted, he prepares cages and bedding for them. He then cleans the animal housing area, does laundry, and cleans equipment used by the

(continued on the next page)

(continued from the previous page)

vets. A client brings in a stray kitten she found. It is still at an age where it is nursing and cannot eat solid foot yet. While the veterinary assistant calls the shelter they work with to find someone to foster the kitten, José prepares formula and bottle-feeds it. At the end of his shift, he again walks the dogs before going home. Not all aspects of his job are pleasant, but José enjoys working with animals.

in urban and suburban areas. They usually treat pets, most commonly cats and dogs. However, rabbits, reptiles, snakes, and birds are also brought to these kinds of practices.

Large animal practices are found mostly in rural areas. These practices treat farm animals, including cows, horses, sheep, and pigs. They may also treat animals such as alpacas, bred for their fur, and, in some cases, poultry such as chickens. Veterinarians and their assistants in large animal practices often assist in the birth of farm animals when they are having difficulty. Large animal practice assistants must be physically strong, have great stamina, and be willing to work outdoors in inclement weather. Large animal practices provide very important support to farmers and ranchers, who depend on their animals for their livelihood. Mixed-practice vets treat both large and small animals. Such practices are common in small towns in rural areas, where there may be only one veterinary practice.

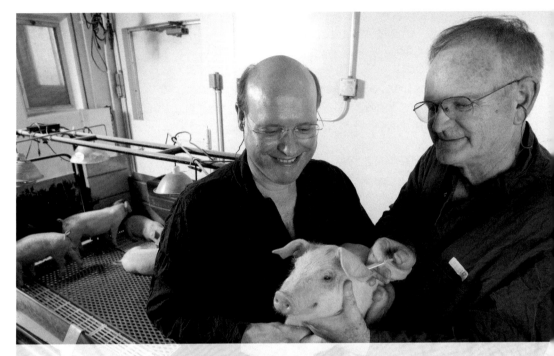

A veterinary technician helps a veterinarian vaccinate a young pig so that it doesn't get sick. Rural veterinarian practices help farmers keep their livestock healthy.

Exotic animal practices specialize in animals other than common pets. They may treat birds, reptiles and snakes, or small mammals other than cats and dogs, including injured wildlife such as squirrels and foxes.

Mobile veterinary services make house calls, treating animals in clients' homes. They typically have a van containing the equipment they need and often employ an assistant who travels with them.

Veterinary offices are often closed in the evenings and on weekends, providing staff with a regular work schedule. If animals are kept on-site, an animal care attendant will care for the animals in the evenings and on weekends. Animal hospitals treat animals that require major surgery or have serious illnesses. Often cases requiring advanced care are referred by veterinary offices to the hospital. They are open twenty-four hours a day, seven days a week, and provide emergency care at times when regular veterinary practices are closed.

Veterinary assistants and animal care attendants are employed by veterinarians who practice at a variety of other facilities as well. Small animal shelters often work with a local veterinary practice that provides the services they need. However, large organizations may have their

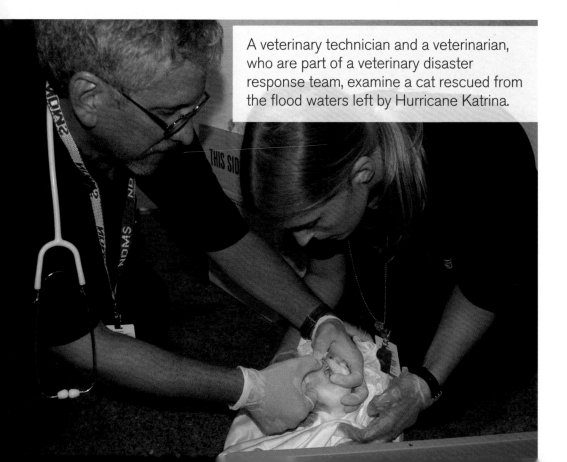

A veterinary technician and a veterinarian, who are part of a veterinary disaster response team, examine a cat rescued from the flood waters left by Hurricane Katrina.

own veterinary staff. Animal rehabilitation facilities treat and house injured wildlife and, when possible, return them to the wild. Animal sanctuaries provide a home for wild animals that cannot be returned to the wild. Animal preserves are open, parklike or wild areas of land on which wildlife is allowed to roam freely, living in the wild but protected from poachers and hunters. Equine veterinarians and staff work at racetracks and horse breeding farms to care for the horses. Zoos, aquariums, and animal parks, such as Busch Gardens, Disney's Animal Park, and SeaWorld, also employ a veterinary staff. They not only treat injured or sick animals but also play a key role in preventing disease in healthy animals. Often, animal preserves and animal parks are involved in breeding programs designed to repopulate endangered species. Wildlife veterinarians and their staff play a key role in these programs. As can be seen, employment in the veterinary field gives one the opportunity to work with the type and size of animal one prefers. It also allows one to work in the setting of one's choice—urban, rural, or the wild.

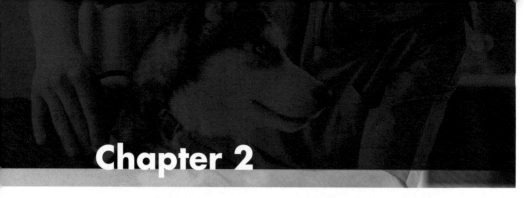

Chapter 2

CLINICAL JOBS IN VETERINARY MEDICINE

There are various types of veterinary jobs available for high school graduates that require two years or less of training. For each of the jobs described here, information will be provided on educational and training requirements, tasks, equipment and technology used, responsibilities, and work environments.

Animal Care Associates and Attendants

Animal care associates (also called animal care attendants) provide the daily care for inpatient animals at veterinary facilities. They clean cages, feed animals, and exercise them. In addition, they monitor the health of the animals and report any changes to the veterinarian. These attendants also keep the facility clean and maintain records. This position requires only a high school diploma or general equivalency degree (GED), and it can be full- or part-time, which offers the opportunity to work while attending school and taking courses for a more advanced position.

Veterinary Assistants and Technicians

Veterinary assistants help veterinarians evaluate and treat animals. The term "veterinary assistant" is used in different contexts. Some practices use the term to refer to the individuals who handle some animal care responsibilities and assist with basic clinical tasks, such as holding animals during exams and cleaning equipment. This type of assistant position requires only a high school

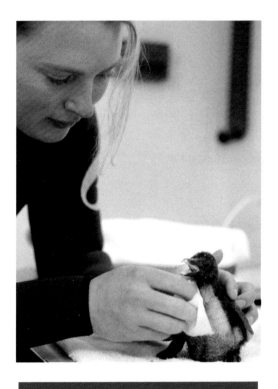

An animal care specialist wipes the face of a penguin chick after feeding it at an aquarium.

diploma and hands-on animal care experience. In other practices, the term is used synonymously with the term "veterinary technician."

Certified veterinary assistants and certified veterinary technicians have completed a two-year associate's degree program and passed a certification exam, such as that offered by the National Association of Veterinary Technicians in America (NAVTA). Animal hospitals, which often perform surgery and treat seriously ill animals, generally prefer certified veterinary technicians. Veterinary technicians handle animals during examinations, collect samples for laboratory analysis, give medication, operate equipment, give injections and vaccinations, assist veterinarians during surgery, and keep records.

Veterinary assistants or technicians in a large animal practice travel to farms or ranches with a veterinarian. They help veterinarians catch animals such as cows, pigs, sheep, goats, and horses and hold them so that they can be treated. They help in the delivery of calves and other

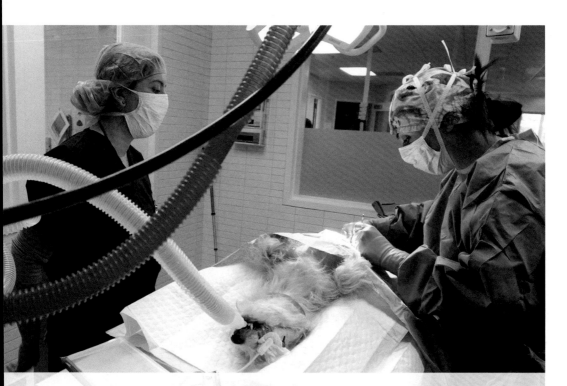

A certified veterinary assistant at an ASPCA shelter assists a veterinarian who is spaying a dog to prevent her from having litters of puppies and adding to the population of stray dogs.

animals when the mother is having difficulty delivering on her own. They prepare syringes for injections, help with cleaning wounds, and perform other tasks as necessary. Being a large animal assistant requires great physical strength and determination, because the job requires handling big, heavy animals that are often determined to get away. The job involves working outdoors in all types of weather.

A typical educational program to become a veterinary technician includes the following subjects:

- Veterinary office etiquette and hospital procedures
- Animal restraint
- Examination room procedures
- Pharmacy and pharmacology
- Surgical preparation and assisting
- Small animal nursing
- Laboratory procedures
- Radiology (X-rays) and ultrasound (sound wave) imaging
- Pet cardiopulmonary resuscitation (CPR) and first aid certification
- The student also performs a hundred hours of onsite hands-on clinical work.

At the time of this writing, NAVTA, the organization that certifies veterinary technicians, is undertaking the Veterinary Nurse Initiative. The purpose of the initiative is to change the title, certification, and licensing for skilled veterinary assistants with associate's or bachelor's degrees. Instead of veterinary technicians, NAVTA would designate them as veterinary nurses. There would be

A certified veterinary technician positions a dog while a veterinarian performs an ultrasound scan of its stomach. Certified veterinary technicians often assist in technical procedures.

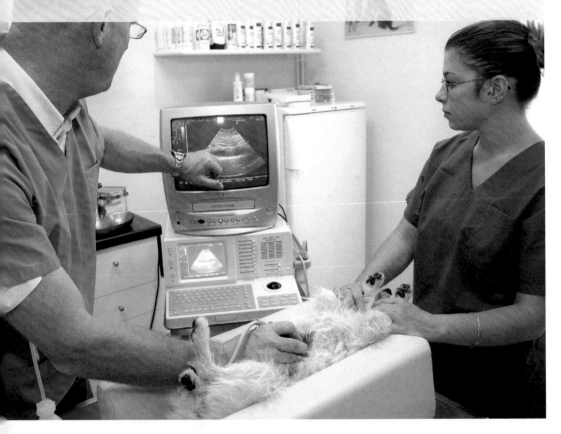

several benefits from the name change. First, the term "veterinary nurse" emphasizes the responsibility for animal care, not just the technical side of the job. Second, it clarifies the difference between veterinary technicians, who have at least an associate's degree, and noncollege-graduate assistants who perform less technical tasks but may also be called "veterinary assistants." Once NAVTA has achieved the required legal changes to state licensing laws, the organization plans to offer two levels of veterinary nurse certification: registered veterinary nurse (RVN)

A DAY IN THE LIFE OF A VETERINARY ASSISTANT

Melissa's first task each day is to make sure that everything is ready in the patient treatment and surgery areas. She checks that there are adequate supplies of bandages, bedding, and medical supplies. She checks the surgery schedule and makes sure the operating room is clean and set up for the first patient.

Once the practice opens for the day, Melissa helps the veterinarians by restraining animals during examinations. When an animal needs an X-ray or a magnetic resonance imaging (MRI) scan, she positions and holds the animal for the veterinary technician. When an animal needs surgery, she clips and shaves the area where the surgery will be done, then removes the loose fur and cleans the area. After the animal has been transported to the operating room, she cleans all the equipment in the preparation area so that it is safe for the next animal.

During routine procedures in the examining room, Melissa helps the veterinarians by providing the material and equipment they need. She handles puppies and kittens

(continued on the next page)

(continued from the previous page)

coming in for their first vaccinations, restrains a cat that doesn't want its nails clipped, and holds injured animals so the veterinarian can examine and treat their wounds. At the end of a long day, she makes sure that all the tools are sterilized and the equipment is clean and prepared for the next day.

for veterinary nurses with an associate's degree and BSVN for those who have a bachelor's degree. (There is also a certification credential planned for MSVN, for veterinary nurses with a master's degree.)

Veterinary Receptionist

The veterinary receptionist checks in animals, communicates with owners, keeps records, orders supplies, bills customers, and collects payments. The American Animal Hospital Association (AAHA) provides a certification program for veterinary receptionists. It offers the Veterinary Receptionist Certificate course online. Many veterinary receptionists go on to become veterinary assistants or technicians or veterinary practice managers. This job requires only a high school diploma, but bookkeeping skills and a knowledge of software used in businesses are helpful. Those interested in becoming a veterinary receptionist should learn common word processing and spreadsheet programs or take a high school business vocational program if one is offered.

Veterinary Lab Assistants

Veterinary lab assistants help the laboratory technicians with testing of blood, tissue, and other bodily samples to diagnose diseases of animals. They enter data into the laboratory information system (LIS), check in samples, and email, fax, and phone results to veterinarians who order tests.

They prepare samples for analysis within the lab or for shipping to outside facilities. They fill supply orders and assist with testing. This position requires only a high school diploma or GED. With additional education and experience, lab assistants can advance to the position of lab technician, performing the tests themselves.

Gaining Necessary Experience

Although a large number of jobs exist for students with just a high school diploma, most listings say "at least one year of veterinary or animal care experience required." Therefore, it helps to gain animal care experience while in high school by performing part-time paid or volunteer work at an animal shelter, animal rescue or rehabilitation facility, or kennel. When such work is performed for a privately run animal sanctuary or an animal rescue organization, it not only provides experience for the student but also helps these nonprofit organizations, which usually cannot afford to hire large numbers of staff and often have a great deal of work to

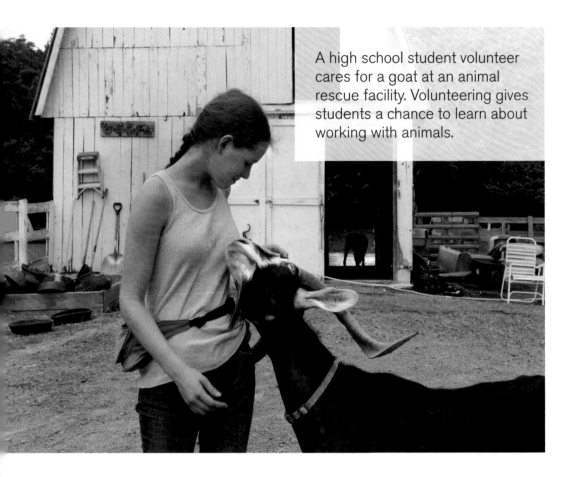

A high school student volunteer cares for a goat at an animal rescue facility. Volunteering gives students a chance to learn about working with animals.

contend with. In this way, volunteering helps the entire community.

Being Successful in Veterinary Care

The following qualities will help one succeed as an animal care associate, veterinary assistant, or veterinary technician. Those in veterinary support positions must have strong listening skills, so that they are certain to understand and correctly follow veterinarians' instructions.

They must be attentive to detail and have good observational skills, so as to note subtle changes in animals' conditions that might need to be addressed. They must care about animals and be calm and patient with them. Sometimes animals will be frightened—they may bite or scratch, or, in the case of large animals, run and hide or be hard to catch. Those who care for animals must be able to deal with uncooperative animals, upset clients, and situations in which they can't help an animal. Despite these frustrations, they must put the animal's welfare first. Animal care staff must be able to solve problems. Sometimes an off-the-shelf solution to an injured animal's situation doesn't exist, and they must be able to come up with options and evaluate them to arrive at the one most likely to work. They must also be flexible. If one approach won't work, they must adjust and try something else. They must be willing to work long hours or outside of regular working hours when necessary. Veterinary care offers many positive interactions with animals, including the opportunity to handle healthy (and adorable) puppies and kittens receiving routine care. However, sometimes the staff will have to deal with animals that have been abused or that need to be euthanatized because they are beyond treatment. Animal care professionals must be able to deal emotionally with such situations.

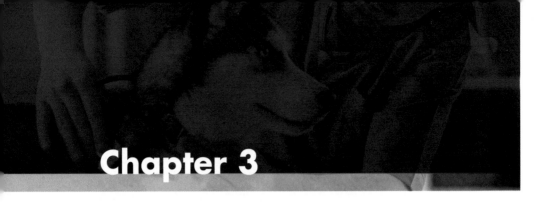

Chapter 3

RELATED JOBS

There are numerous jobs caring for and protecting animals aside from clinical jobs at veterinary clinics and hospitals. Public and private animal sanctuaries and shelters, wild animal preserves, state and national parks, and zoos and aquariums all offer employment opportunities for those interested in an animal care career.

Kennel and Shelter Attendants

Kennel and shelter attendants provide daily care for the animals that are boarded in a kennel or housed at an animal shelter. They schedule appointments, clean cages and dog runs, and bathe, groom, exercise, and feed animals. They administer medication and monitor the behavior and health of the animals. There are no particular educational requirements for this job. So it is a good part-time as well as full-time job for high-school and college students and can provide the experience needed to get a higher-level veterinary job. Many attendants go on to become kennel or shelter managers or open their own grooming, pet-sitting, boarding, or doggie day-care business.

Animal Caretaker

Animal caretakers provide care for animals in zoos and aquariums. Their major responsibilities are preparing food for the animals, feeding them, and cleaning their habitats. They observe the animals under their care to make sure they are healthy. One of the main focuses of animal parks, preserves, zoos, and aquariums today is to breed endangered species. If they are successful, then it is common for the female to be monitored by the veterinary staff throughout her preg-

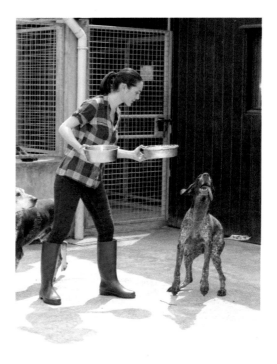

An animal care attendant feeds dogs at an animal shelter. Shelter attendants keep the animals' cages clean and bathe, groom, and comfort animals.

nancy to make sure she and the babies are healthy. Mothers may be checked onsite or brought to the veterinary station for checkups. After the birth, if there are problems, such as the mother refusing to nurse or having too many offspring to care for, one or more babies may be brought to the veterinary station, where they are fed, cared for, and played with by the staff until they are old

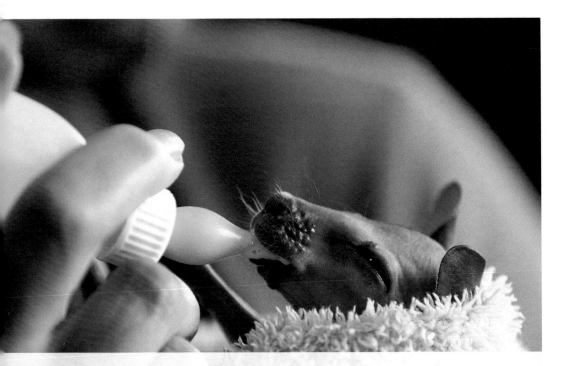

An animal caretaker at a zoo bottle-feeds a baby wallaby. Ensuring the survival of every baby born to an endangered species is a priority.

enough to be released into the general population. Animals with physical problems will also be treated by the veterinary staff.

Some large zoos and aquariums also participate in animal rescue operations. The rescued animals are then treated by the veterinary staff at the facility. Animal caretaker positions generally require only a high school diploma or GED. Zoos and aquariums that have onsite veterinary departments employ veterinary technicians whose responsibilities are similar to those of veterinary

WORKING AS A WILDLIFE TECHNICIAN

The story of a student working on a study conducted by the Canadian Wildlife Health Cooperative presents an example of one type of activity performed by wildlife technicians. Over one summer, Collin Letain began each morning by checking wire traps set up at the Indi, Barber, and Rice Lakes in the Canadian province of Saskatchewan. The traps were funnel-shaped with a wide opening at one end. When a duck swam in, it was unable to swim out again. Letain removed any trapped ducks, including American Wigeon, Blue and Green Winged Teal, Gadwall, Mallard, Northern Pintail, and Northern Shoveler ducks. He then placed an identification band around the leg of any adult ducks to allow their migratory pattern to be tracked. There was another purpose to trapping the ducks, however—a health concern. Letain swabbed each duck's throat. The swabs were taken back to the laboratory and tested for avian flu. Thus far, no flu has been found, but if it were to develop, it would represent a threat to the poultry raised in the United States and

(continued on the next page)

(continued from the previous page)

Canada and to people. When all the birds had been banded and released, Letain reset the traps, baiting them with barley, so they would be ready for the next day. His work in assisting the CWHC to make sure ducks were healthy helped protect the animals they survey, domestic animals, and people in the United States and Canada.

technicians in other types of practices. To be hired as a veterinary technician in a zoo or aquarium, one must have completed a veterinary technician program and be certified or licensed by the state in which one practices. Large zoos might have various grades of technicians, whose responsibilities increase with their level of training.

Wildlife Technician

Wildlife technicians help biologists and game officers manage and preserve wildlife and their habitats. They work in wildlife preserves, state parks, and related facilities. The majority are employed by state fish and game departments or by the federal government. They frequently help with research projects, trapping and tagging animals, providing care for captured animals, collecting biological specimens, observing and counting animal populations, entering data for evaluation, maintaining and calibrating scientific equipment, and writing reports. Most entry-level wildlife technician jobs require a two-year associate's degree in wildlife biology, ecology, zoology, animal science, or a related area. The activities of a wildlife technician include some or all of the following: They collect biological samples in the field. They might set traps for a certain type of animal and then take a sample of blood or saliva to test for disease. They then usually band or tag the animal before releasing it so that the same animal is not tested more than once.

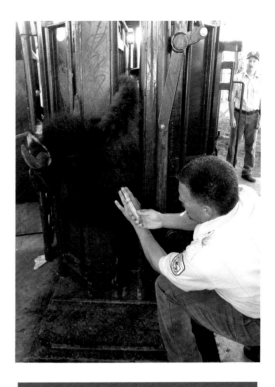

A wildlife technician draws blood from a bison at a wildlife preserve to check for any health problems that could affect the animal or the herd.

They also participate in ground- or air-based surveys of animal populations. In ground-based surveys, technicians might walk to particular points in the area being surveyed and record the number of animals of one or more species they observe there. In some cases, they stake out a specific location and record the population of animals there. For example, a national park in Canada built a concrete bridge over the highway crossing the park to allow animals to avoid the auto traffic. A technician might be sent to a spot in the brush near the overpass to observe how many animals use it and how well they negotiate it. The results of the survey could be used in a study to decide whether or not to build such walkways at other national parks. Aerial wildlife surveys are conducted from a helicopter or small plane. The purpose is the same—to locate and count wildlife, and sometimes to monitor the traveling of herds. Technicians also enter survey data into computers and use computer programs to compile and analyze the data. They might prepare charts and tables for inclusion in reports.

Technicians also check and repair structures, and maintain equipment used by the team. For example, cameras are often set up overnight to catch pictures of

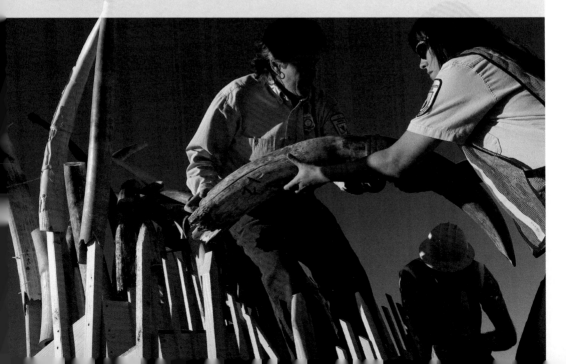

A wildlife inspector and a technician for the US Fish and Wildlife Service prepare confiscated illegal ivory from African and Asian elephants for destruction.

animals traversing a particular area. The technician would check the cameras each day to make sure they are operating properly. As technicians undertake additional education and gain experience, they can move up to more senior wildlife technician positions and supervisory positions, and into positions such as wildlife inspector. Wildlife inspectors monitor shipments of imported and exported animals to ensure compliance with the laws. They also review shipments for products made from wildlife, including leather shoes and bags, furs, and trophies.

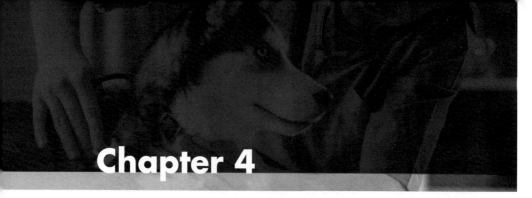

Chapter 4

LEARNING TO CARE FOR ANIMALS

The education required for veterinary jobs ranges from on-the-job training to programs that take several months to two years. There are various sources of training programs, including online programs, community colleges, and conventional colleges. However, the fact that many entry-level jobs require only a high school diploma does not mean that no preparation is required. One can increase one's chances of getting a job both by preparing academically and by gaining practical experience while in school.

During High School

Whether one is planning to go directly to work after high school or take additional academic training, it is essential to gain a basic understanding of math and science while in high school. This necessity is particularly important for those planning to apply for work directly after completing high school, because this background will assure employers that one can master the skills required for the job.

Veterinary work requires a lot of math. If one wants to be a veterinary or wildlife assistant or technician (or to advance to such a position from an entry-level animal care job), it will be necessary to have a good grasp of math. In those jobs one has to calculate dosages of medications and perform calculations when evaluating test results and calibrating test equipment. A knowledge of biology and chemistry provides a solid foundation for understanding animal anatomy and health. Veterinary technicians and lab assistants work with many types of equipment. A knowledge of physics can help them understand how such machines—as well as parts of the body—function.

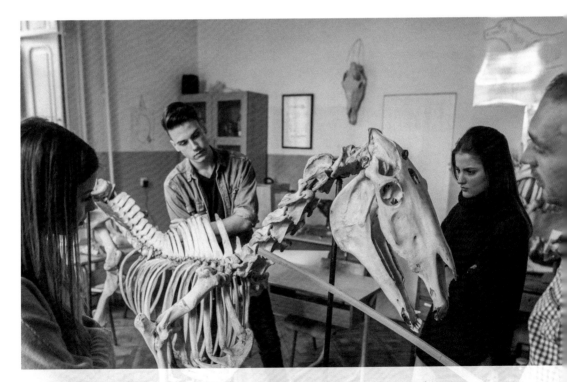

Students study the skeleton of a horse. Students interested in veterinary careers benefit from learning about the anatomy of animals while in high school.

An option for students who do not plan to attend college is a high school vocational program. Many towns and cities offer such practical training courses, and many have dedicated technical vocational high schools. Some of these vocational high schools, such as the Worcester Technical High School in Worcester, Massachusetts, offer programs in veterinary assisting. The program provides practical and academic training designed to prepare students to work as veterinary assistants in different settings. The program provides hands-on training at an on-site veterinary clinic and prepares students to take the national certification exam to become an Approved Veterinary Assistant. Students who complete this program graduate job-ready and with hands-on experience. If one is interested in starting in a veterinary receptionist or shelter clerk position, it is worth considering entering a vocational high school program in business. This type of program provides one with a knowledge of the major software programs that are used in offices and often offers training in areas such as billing and bookkeeping, which are in demand in veterinary practices.

Although many people view veterinary careers as "dealing with animals," in most cases they involve a great deal of interaction with people. Veterinary staff at all levels must deal with clients to arrange and provide care for their animals. Often, people are upset and worried about their pets, so excellent communication skills are a plus. In addition, veterinary staff must record information about animals under their care. Those working with wild-life will be part of a team, and communicating observations and writing reports will be part of their job. For these reasons, it is important to communicate well with both patients and staff members, both in writing and verbally. If your school offers a course in public speaking, taking it can help you hone your skills for addressing members of the public. When communicating with clients and other team members, it is important that your meaning and information be understood correctly. Therefore, it is necessary to learn the rules of English grammar and the ways to convey information accurately and avoid misunderstandings.

In veterinary positions, staff members constantly use computers—to enter and transmit patient data, check an animal's history, compile and analyze data, and write reports. Those working as assistants and receptionists in veterinary practices or as assistants and technicians in wildlife programs will have to learn the organization's special software programs, whether they are analyzing data, entering test results, or maintaining patient records and doing billing. So, if your school offers computer training, take advantage of it. Computer technology changes

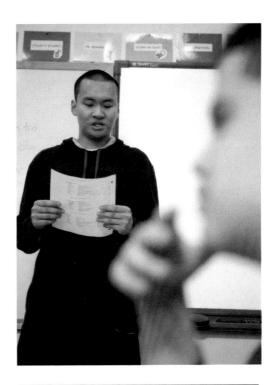

A student gives a speech in class. Learning how to communicate clearly and effectively will make a person a better team member and reduce misunderstandings.

constantly—the better you understand the principles, the easier you'll find it to learn new programs and technologies. Likewise, if your school offers a typing or keyboarding course, it's beneficial to take it.

Learning at least one language other than English can help you better communicate with clients and, in some cases, other team members. This knowledge is also an advantage when applying for a job, especially in locations where there is a large population that speaks another language, such as Spanish or French. Which language will be most beneficial depends on the population of the area in which you live or would like to practice. The most commonly spoken languages other than English in the United States and Canada are Spanish, French, Russian, Arabic, and Chinese.

Volunteering and Internships

The major difficulty job seekers face is competing against more experienced candidates for their first job. Having previous experience assures employers that they can perform the required tasks. This background is vital in jobs that require people to handle animals, for the safety of both the animals and those caring for them. Nonprofit organizations such as animal shelters, animal rescue organizations, and animal rehabilitation facilities often need volunteers. One can call or visit such facilities to check out available opportunities. Some large organizations, such as the Humane Society and the National Park Service, post information about volunteering on their website. If you live in a rural area or are interested in a position in a large animal practice, it's worth participating

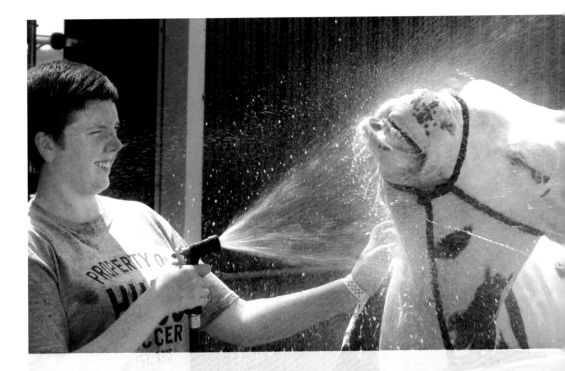

A teenager competing at a 4-H fair hoses down her cow. Learning to handle and care for animals properly will help in veterinary work later.

in 4-H programs. Young people in these programs raise farm animals and participate in competitions with them.

Another way to gain experience is through an internship at a company. Internships are usually unpaid positions that allow a student to learn on-the-job skills. Facilities may have internship positions open to high school students, to high school graduates, or both. Interns carry out basic tasks that support the veterinary team, such as feeding animals, walking dogs, cleaning cages, and entering data. They not only gain experience in the activities they perform but also learn how to work as part of an animal care team. Both aspects are important to employers. Although interns do not typically perform advanced activities, they have the opportunity to observe and learn how those tasks are done. Internships often give students a chance to become familiar with the protocols and software used in veterinary work. When students are in college, internships give them an opportunity to see how the tools and techniques they learn about in school are used in the real world. Internships also provide a chance to develop contacts with professionals in the field, which can help when looking for a job. First, if someone does a good job as an intern, it's possible to obtain a reference that can be used when looking for a first real job. Second, if someone is working at a large facility and a position opens up, he or she might be offered a job. Third, many veterinary staff members obtain their first job as the result of personal contacts, especially in wildlife and zoo work. Even if a permanent job is not available at the facility where a student interns, the people he or she works with might be able to recommend him or her to others who are looking for an employee. There are many resources available that provide information on veterinary internships. It's common for general job listing sites such as CareerBuilder.com to list such positions. One can do a search on "veterinary internship" to see available positions. Websites for individual animal hospitals, clinics, parks, zoos, and aquariums often have a "jobs" or "careers" link, which includes openings for interns. Professional organizations, such as the National Association of Veterinary Technicians, often list openings for interns on their website as well. Students should also

A DAY IN THE LIFE OF A VETERINARY TECHNICIAN

Lindsay Calhoun works at an emergency animal hospital as a licensed veterinary technician. She explained her day-to-day tasks in an interview with Sara Royster that was published in the *Occupational Outlook Quarterly*. Calhoun works in different parts of the hospital and always has to do such tasks as clean out the animal cages, thoroughly clean exam and operating tables, sterilize equipment, and clean up after the animals.

When she is assigned to the operating room, she prepares the animal, begins the intravenous drip feed, and watches the anesthesia that is required during the procedure. When she is scheduled to work in the treatment room, she cares for all the animals, including the preoperative preparation. During the day, she might have to give animals their medications, depending on their illnesses. She also tries to give them all loving attention. Because emergency animal hospitals are usually hectic, Calhoun sometimes helps in the lab, spinning tubes of urine or blood, sending out blood work, or looking at slides using a microscope. Some days,

(continued on the next page)

(continued from the previous page)

Calhoun works with the appointments that don't need the veterinarian that have been scheduled for the day. In these cases, she gives vaccines, changes bandages, or removes stitches.

Calhoun enjoys working in animal emergency medicine and plans to volunteer when possible to help animal shelters. Her advice for people who are thinking of pursuing veterinary technician careers is the following:

Go through school and get your license ... you'll have more job options and be able to earn more money ... I think it's important to get a job in an animal hospital as soon as you can ... It doesn't matter if you don't have any practical experience yet. Apply to work in the kennel to get your foot in the door ... Hands-on experience, along with the knowledge you will get in school, will make you a better veterinary technician.

Calhoun says that her daily experiences with all kinds of animals throughout her life provided an ideal starting point for pursuing a job in an animal hospital.

contact the veterinary facilities in the area where they live and ask if there are any openings for an intern. Some colleges offer a program that includes 100 to 240 hours of practical training in a veterinary clinic as part of the educational program. This school-arranged internship is referred to as an "externship."

One advantage of volunteering or becoming an intern is that it gives a person a chance to develop a relationship with an experienced veterinary professional who can act as a mentor. Having a mentor can help people develop leadership skills faster and avoid mistakes. A mentor can also be a source of advice and support when a person is starting out in the field. If a staff member mentors you, it is important to show your gratitude and thank him or her for the help.

Veterinary Certificate Training Programs

For the student who does not participate in a veterinary assistant vocational course in high school, the alternative is to take a veterinary assistant certificate training program after graduation. Such programs are available at community colleges, technical schools, and online. They generally take one year to complete. Regardless of whether people choose a physical or online program, it is important to make sure that it is NVTA-approved, so that they can take the national Approved Veterinary Assistant certification test upon completing the program. Although certification is not required in many states, certification gives people an advantage in the job search. Many facilities prefer to hire certified veterinary assistants, so as to be sure that they have the required skills. In addition, certified veterinary assistants generally receive higher salaries than noncertified ones.

Veterinary certification programs typically cover the following subjects:

- Animal anatomy, physiology, and terminology
- Math fundamentals
- Computer basics
- First aid and CPR
- Clinical laboratory tests and procedures
- Pathology (disease processes)
- Office practices
- Students also participate in an externship.

Associate's Degree Programs

If one wants to work as a veterinary technician, it will be necessary to take a two-year associate's degree course. Like certificate programs, associate's degree programs are provided online and at technical schools, community colleges, and traditional colleges and universities. Taking the program at a four-year school often allows one to complete a bachelor's degree later with another two years of academic training at the same school.

If one is taking an associate's degree course online, it's essential to ensure that the school is accredited. This confirmation makes certain that the degree is valid and that the credits earned can be transferred to another school if one decides to pursue a bachelor's degree later. Check for accreditation at the US Department of Education's database of accredited postsecondary institutions (https://ope.ed.gov/accreditation).

The veterinary technology curriculum is very detailed and often requires a certain number of observation hours within a veterinary hospital. Some programs require students to complete externships or internships to acquire the necessary field training. The overall coursework for a veterinarian technician program includes all the courses in a typical veterinarian assistant certificate program plus biochemistry, animal pharmacology, the diagnosis and treatment of animal diseases, veterinary nursing, surgical assisting, and veterinary dentistry, among other courses.

In some states, veterinary technicians must pass a licensing exam. Most states use the Veterinary Technician National Exam (VTNE) from the American Association of

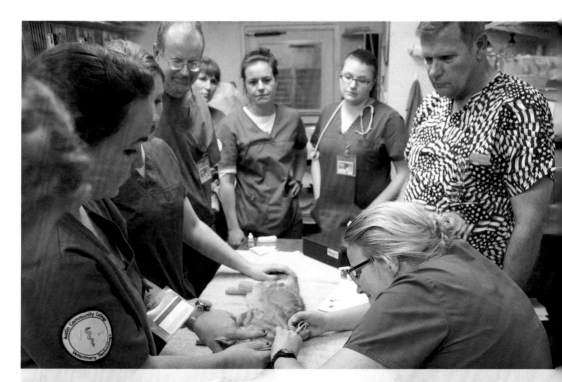

Veterinary students position a cat for examination. They help with worming, testing, and caring for animals as part of their practical training.

Veterinary State Boards for licensing purposes. It consists of two hundred multiple-choice questions that must be answered within four hours. Check with your state licensing board of veterinary medicine to find the requirements in your state.

To become a wildlife technician, one must have an associate's degree in applied science. Some online and physical colleges offer associate's degrees in wildlife technology. In such a program, students take courses in areas including the following:

- Biology
- Terrestrial wildlife management
- Wetlands and fisheries wildlife management
- Statistics
- Animal identification
- First aid and CPR
- Forestry
- Aerial photography interpretation
- English composition and speech

Students learn the use of the various types of equipment and computer programs used in the field. Physical colleges sometimes include a combination of classroom and outdoor fieldwork. In this case, students might perform work in zoos, state parks, fisheries, and lakes.

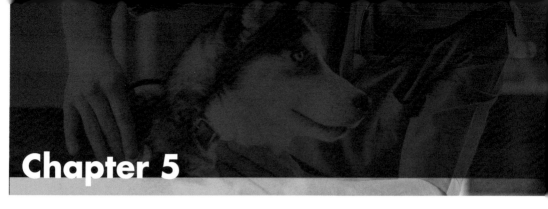

Chapter 5

LANDING A VETERINARY JOB

Whether one goes directly into a position that provides on-the-job training or takes a certificate or associate's degree program, the next step is to find a job. This section discusses how to locate and obtain an entry-level veterinary job and how to maximize one's chances of success in the field.

Creating a Résumé

To apply for a job you need a résumé. The résumé's function is to convince a potential employer to interview you. It describes your skills, experience, and training. Focus your résumé on the specific skills required for the job you are applying for, to make yourself a more attractive candidate. It is simple to keep a master résumé on your computer and modify it as needed to emphasis the skills and experience called for in a job ad.

There are many formats for a résumé, but for an entry-level job, it's best to use a simple, easy-to-follow format. Start with your personal information, including name,

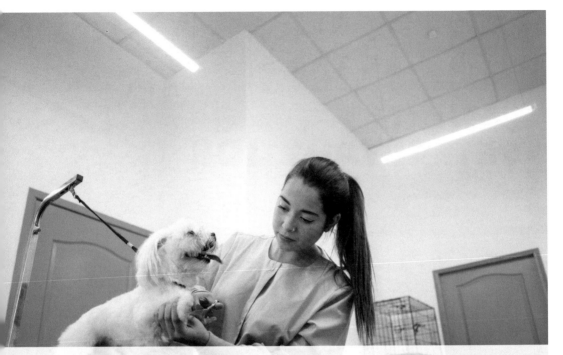

A high-school student grooms a dog at a pet store. The weekend job in the store provides her with experience working with animals, which she can include on her résumé.

address, cell phone number, and email address. Next, list your previous employment, starting with the most recent. You should include all part-time jobs, summer jobs, and volunteer, internship, and externship positions you have had, including non-veterinary jobs where you used relevant skills, such as working in a pet shop (even if you were a clerk) or earning money by walking dogs.

Next, list your education, including any relevant vocational program in high school or certificate or degree programs you've completed, and any certifications or licenses you have received. If you are applying for a job straight from high school without formal training, provide a list of relevant courses taken in high school, such as biology, chemistry, physics, or computer courses, and any vocational courses that provide medical or technical skills.

There are a great many non-English-speaking patients and staff in animal care and medicine. Therefore, if you are fluent in a language other than English, mention this expertise on your résumé as well. Being bilingual can be a major advantage when applying for a job, especially in areas with a large population of non-English-speakers.

Proofread your résumé carefully, then have someone else read it over, too. When you are working with sick and injured animals, equipment, and medications, being precisely accurate and paying attention to details are critical. An error can be damaging to an animal and devastating to its owner. Accordingly, you do not want to give a potential employer the impression that you are careless or sloppy by sending a résumé that contains mistakes.

Finding Potential Jobs

There are a variety of ways to locate potential jobs. If you graduate from a program at a college or technical school, the school may have a job placement office. The office not only helps students find jobs but also often assists them in preparing a résumé and developing good interviewing techniques. A major factor in obtaining a veterinary job—especially large animal, zoo, and wildlife positions—is networking. You should contact people you have worked with during internships and externships to

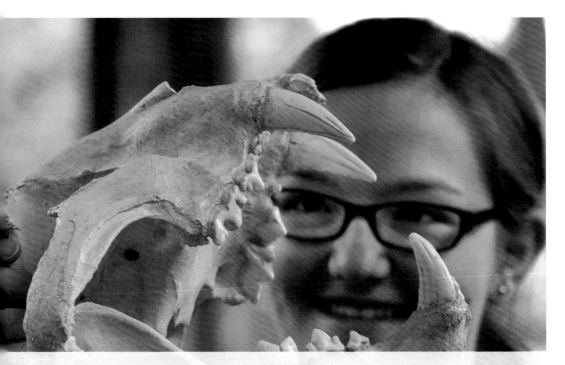

A student intern at a zoo educates visitors about the anatomy of tigers. Animal-related summer jobs and internships provide valuable résumé material and professional contacts.

see if they know of any openings in the field. Even if there are no openings at the facility where you worked, these contacts may be able to tell you of other facilities looking for staff or pass along your résumé or contact information to staff at other institutions.

The other common way to locate potential work is through online resources. You should consult general sites such as Monster.com, CareerBuilder.com, Indeed.com, and the like. These sites provide listings for veterinary jobs as well as for other industries. Zoos, theme parks, state and national parks, and veterinary hospitals and

A DAY IN THE LIFE OF AN EQUINE VETERINARY TECHNICIAN

Samantha Rowland is an equine veterinary technician and a graduate of Wilson College. On Wilson College's website, she described what her job entails. Like most equine veterinarians, her employer has a mobile practice. Rowland is on the road all day, riding to farm calls in a van. Samantha assists in any way necessary. Her job requires holding and handling horses during exams and procedures. Horses are not always easy to handle; they are large and strong animals, and they can be particularly difficult when frightened or injured. They need to be restrained so the veterinarian can treat them. Rowland may also need to walk or trot a horse for a soundness exam. Her other duties include assisting in taking X-rays or ultrasound scans. She helps administer electrical stimulation treatments, draws blood for lab tests, and gives injections.

The hours worked by equine veterinary technicians can be long, sometimes requiring them to attend emergencies late at night or before dawn. Not all equine veterinary

(continued on the next page)

(continued from the previous page)

technicians work with mobile vets. Some equine vet techs care for horses at specialized veterinary hospitals or work at racetracks or breeding farms. Equine veterinary technicians must have good observational skills, so as to notice changes in a horse's movement or attitude. In particular, they must notice any signs of lameness or illness and report them to the veterinarian immediately. To be an equine vet tech, one must also be strong and in good physical health. Because equine veterinary technicians occasionally need to ride a horse, the ability to ride is a necessary skill as well.

veterinary practices—especially large ones with multiple branches—maintain a list of job openings on their websites. Usually these can be accessed through a Jobs or Careers link. Professional organizations for veterinary assistants and veterinary technicians also often list job openings on their websites, allow résumé postings, and send out job alerts when new positions are uploaded.

Many jobs, especially those at the entry level, are not advertised. Therefore, you might find a position by doing cold mailings. This approach means that you look up the veterinary facilities in your area and mail them a hard copy of your résumé with a short cover letter explaining the type of job you are interested in and your qualifications. Simply checking the online or physical Yellow Pages will provide a list of such facilities. Even if a job is not immediately available, résumés are often kept on file, so you might get a call in the future when a position opens up at that facility. Many large institutions, such as zoos, aquariums, and theme parks, have an employment office, where it is possible to stop by in person and fill out an application for a job.

Interviewing for a Veterinary Job

The goal of an interview is to convince an employer that you will contribute to the veterinary team and be an asset to the organization. Two key factors in making a good impression at an interview are professionalism and preparation. Even if you will be working in jeans and a T-shirt, go to the interview dressed and groomed professionally. Wear neat, clean clothing such as slacks and a shirt for men or a slack suit, dress, or skirt and blouse for women. During the interview, speak respectfully, use correct grammar, greet everyone you are

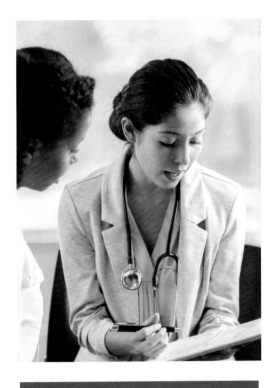

A student practices interview techniques with an instructor. Practice is key to performing well at an interview.

introduced to politely, and address them respectfully. Veterinary staff deal extensively with the public. Therefore, you want to show that you understand that looking and sounding professional is part of your responsibilities.

Preparation for the interview means you understand what the institution does and what is expected of you. Prior to the interview, research the facility on the internet. During the interview you should be able to discuss the particular activities at the facility, what staff members in your position are expected to do, and the skills you have to fill the role required. In the health care field, "people skills" are just as essential as practical skills.

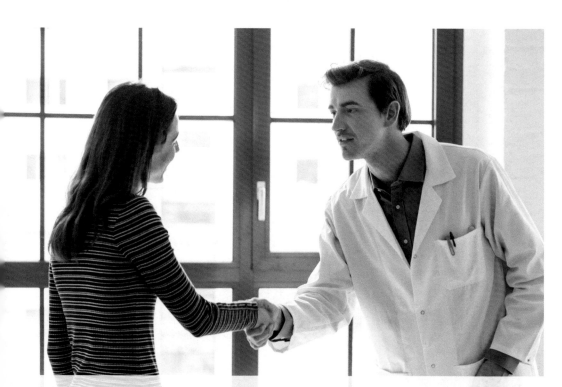

A veterinarian interviews a job applicant. The interview allows the applicant to discuss her experience and demonstrate her knowledge.

Employers are likely to ask questions about why you chose the veterinary field, why you want to work for their facility, what you can offer the organization, what you have accomplished in the past, what your goals are, and what your strengths and weaknesses are. Young people, especially those with little experience, are likely to be asked questions designed to assure the employer that they will be responsible, show up on time, and do their work even when not supervised. These characteristics are especially important in animal care, where staff might be working alone on weekends or evenings, doing important tasks like feeding animals. Come to the interview prepared to give examples that demonstrate your sense of responsibility and reliability. If you are asked about experience or skills that you don't have, express your willingness to learn and explain how your education and previous experience will allow you to develop those skills. After the interview, be sure to thank the interviewer and other staff members you have met.

Chapter 6

PROFESSIONAL DEVELOPMENT AND ADVANCEMENT

A veterinary career offers significant opportunity for advancement. One can progress internally at the organization where one starts working—for example, from animal caretaker to veterinary assistant. Alternately, one can undertake additional education and move on to a higher level of responsibility at the same facility or at another one. One can also use the experience one gains to move into a different type of animal-related work. This section provides information on how to gain additional certifications or degrees through part-time programs as well as the types of jobs available to those who obtain additional education.

Specialty Veterinary Technicians

Training is available for veterinarian technicians to become specialty technicians. The National Association of Veterinary Technicians in America (NAVTA) is the certification authority for specialty technicians. NAVTA offers certification in eleven specialties, as follows:

- **Clinical Pathology Vet Tech.** Clinical pathology vet techs analyze urine or blood samples to diagnose health issues. Certification requirements include four thousand hours or more of experience and two letters of recommendation, plus a case log covering one year and five individual case reports. Applicants must also fill out a skills log.
- **Clinical Practice Vet Tech.** These vet techs work in a particular subspecialty of clinical work: canine or feline, exotic companion animal, or livestock. To achieve certification, one requires at least ten thousand hours of experience, fifty case

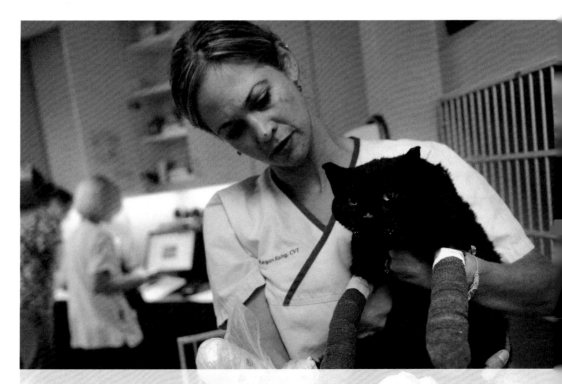

An emergency care veterinary technician prepares to place an injured cat in a cage. Emergency care vet techs often treat animals that have been hurt in accidents.

logs, four case reports, and at least forty hours of continuing education credits.

- **Emergency and Critical Care Vet Tech.** This type of vet tech specializes in treating animals that have been seriously injured or ill. A person who wants to be certified in this specialty needs at least 5,760 hours or more of experience, a case log containing at least fifty cases and covering one year, four detailed case reports, and 25 hours of continuing education.
- **Equine Vet Tech.** These vet techs work with veterinarians who specialize in equine work. They are involved in routine and emergency care for

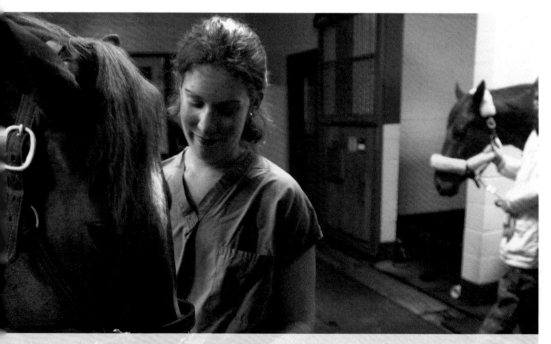

An equine veterinary technician returns a horse to its stall after successful treatment. Being an equine vet tech requires the ability to handle a large animal.

horses. Certification is provided by the American Association of Equine Veterinary Technicians (AAEVT), which offers an online course covering the various aspects of equine care and treatment and the certification exam.

- **Internal Medicine Vet Tech.** Vet techs in the internal medicine specialty work in a particular subspecialty of internal medicine, such as cardiology (heart and blood vessels), neurology (nerves and nervous system), or oncology (cancer). Certification as an internal medicine vet tech requires at least six thousand hours of experience, a case log with fifty to seventy-five cases, four case reports, forty hours of continuing education, two professional letters of recommendation, and a completed skills checklist.

- **Veterinary Behavior Tech.** These vet techs assist in managing and modifying animals' behavior. Being certified requires at least four thousand hours of experience plus either a case log with at least fifty cases or one year of research experience. In either case, applicants must submit five case reports and two letters of recommendation. They must also fill out a checklist of skills and take forty hours of continuing education.

- **Vet Tech Anesthetist.** Vet tech anesthetists assist veterinarian surgeons and anesthesiologists during operations. Among their duties is monitoring sedation and the animal's breathing during the operation. To be certified, one must have six thousand hours of experience, with at least forty-five hundred of those hours working in anesthesia and experience on at least fifty cases during the year in which one applies. One must also complete forty hours of continuing education in the five years prior to submitting an application. Applicants must submit four case reports and two letters of recommendation. They must also fill out a skills checklist.

- **Veterinary Surgical Tech.** Veterinary surgical techs perform preoperative and postoperative activities on animals and assist veterinarians during operations. Certification requires one to have at least ten thousand hours of experience (six thousand hours of which are in the previous three years), with 75 percent of the time spent in surgery.

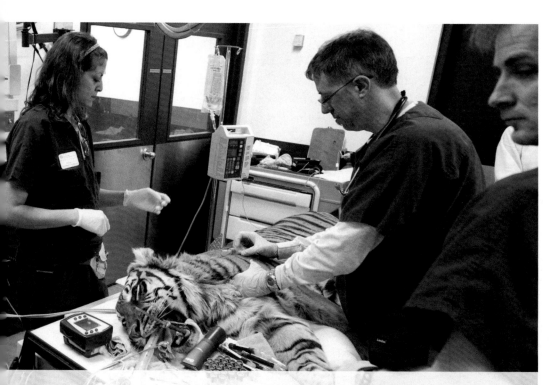

A veterinary technician anesthetist monitors a tiger's sedation while veterinarians work on the animal. It's critical to keep the level of sedation just right.

- **Veterinary Dental Tech.** This type of tech treats dental problems and cleans teeth of animals. Vet dental techs are supervised by a veterinarian. For certification, a person must have at least six thousand hours of experience (at least three thousand hours of which are in dentistry), a case log, five case reports, and forty-one hours of continuing education.
- **Veterinary Nutrition Tech.** These vet techs focus on the management of nutrition for animals. Obtaining certification requires at least four thousand hours of experience in animal nutrition in either a clinical or research setting, two letters of recommendation, forty hours of continuing education, a case log covering one year, and five case reports. Applicants must also either provide evidence of research or complete a skills checklist.
- **Zoo Vet Tech.** These vet techs work with zoo veterinarians treating exotic animals. Being certified as a zoo vet tech requires at least ten thousand hours of experience in zoological veterinary practice, a case log with forty entries, forty hours of continuing education, five case reports, and two letters of recommendation. Applicants must also fill out a skills checklist.

Generally speaking, prior to taking a certification examination, most of the veterinary technician specialists listed need to have accomplished some educational requirements, relevant work experience, animal case logs and reports, and additional continuing education coursework.

RESCUING ANIMALS

Jody Westberg is the head of the team at SeaWorld in Florida that rescues sea mammals. The team retrieves from 250 to 1,000 animals every year. In a *Cosmopolitan* magazine article, she discussed her career in animal care and rescue at SeaWorld. Her experiences not only reveal what working in a major aquarium is like but also illustrate how one can move from an entry-level job to a supervisory position. Her first job at SeaWorld wasn't even in animal care; she worked as an assistant in the accounting department. When she had been there a year, an entry-level job opened up on the team that worked with the park's birds. After several interviews, she won the job. She spent her initial six months working with a mentor, learning how to take care of penguins and their habitat. She then became an official penguin keeper.

From there she decided to move to the entry-level position of husbandry assistant on the mammal department rescue team, which was working to save a whale. Again, she worked with supervisory mentors. The rescue team captures animals, rehabilitates them, and returns them to the wild, if possible. She spent most of her time preparing whale food and observing the mammal team at work. After a year, a higher-level position became available on the rescue team. She learned how to take care of manatees, sea lions, dolphins, and sea otters. In her job, she has to deal with animals that are injured, and about 68 to 72 percent of the rescued animals survive. Hers is not a 9-to-5 job. Animals can require rescuing anytime and any day, including holidays.

In the article, she says, "One of the things I love about my job is every day is different. One day, I'm rescuing a 5-pound [2.3-kilogram] neonatal sea lion pup, and the next day, I'm out responding to a [stranded] juvenile humpback whale that weighs 20,000 pounds [9,072 kg]."

Veterinary Practice Manager

Veterinary practice managers oversee the business aspects of a veterinary practice. Their responsibilities include staff management and scheduling, inventory control, bookkeeping, payroll administration, budgeting, advertising, establishing clinic policies and procedures, training new staff, medical records management, and client relations. Veterinary receptionists who wish to advance to practice management should take courses that provide business management skills such as bookkeeping, budgeting, advertising, and human resource management, among other subjects. Online and physical colleges and community colleges offer one- and two-year certificate programs in business management, or one can enroll in a full- or part-time bachelor's degree program.

Animal Health Inspectors

Animal health inspectors examine facilities that house animals, such as animal shelters, pet stores, and livestock markets. They also check food animal production facilities, feedlots, and fish hatcheries. Research laboratories that use animals in their research are also under their jurisdiction. Animal health inspectors make certain that these operations meet the state and federal regulations for the housing and treatment of animals to ensure that the animals are treated humanely and stay healthy. They help law enforcement investigate reports of unlicensed animal facilities and, if necessary, close them down.

In most cases, animal inspectors have a bachelor's degree in an area such as zoology, veterinary medicine, or animal science, although some start with an associate's degree. State requirements vary, and in some states, they must be licensed veterinary technicians. Most inspectors have previous experience working in a large animal veterinary practice or in livestock management.

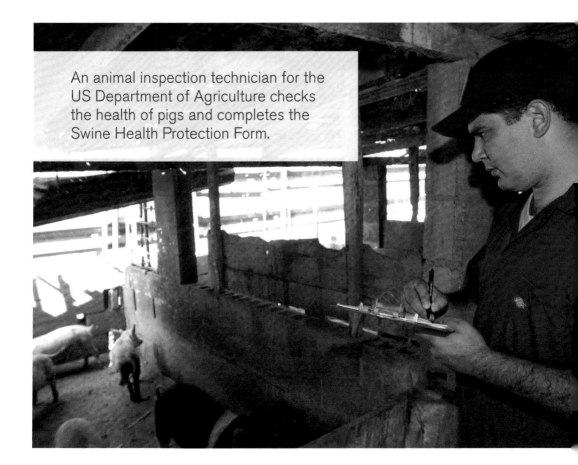

An animal inspection technician for the US Department of Agriculture checks the health of pigs and completes the Swine Health Protection Form.

Wildlife Manager

Wildlife managers oversee all aspects of wildlife conservation and management in a specific territory. They work in animal preserves, state and federal parks, fisheries, and similar areas for protected wildlife. Most work for state fish, game, or wildlife departments or the federal government, although some work for privately owned wildlife preserves. They carry out population surveys of animal species, protect natural resources and endangered species, see that any significant damage to the habitat is repaired, and study the interactions among various species within the territory. They supervise wildlife technicians, wildlife rehabilitators, administrative staff, and volunteers.

Most wildlife managers are required to have a bachelor's degree in wildlife biology, ecology, zoology, animal science, or a similar field. Those seeking jobs with the US Fish and Wildlife Service must have either a bachelor of science degree in biology (or a closely related field) or an equivalent combination of education and experience. Many wildlife managers begin their careers as wildlife technicians or in other related roles to gain the necessary experience.

Conclusion

As has been pointed out, there are many different types of careers related to animal health and care. One of the advantages of a veterinary career is that it is possible to begin at an entry-level position with little training and work one's way up to progressively more responsible positions. Another advantage of this field is that it provides the opportunity to work in the type of setting and with the type of animals one prefers.

GLOSSARY

accredited Officially recognized as maintaining appropriate educational standards, especially for preparing graduates for professional practice.

cardiology The medical discipline that deals with the heart and blood vessels.

cardiopulmonary resuscitation (CPR) An emergency procedure designed to revive a person or animal whose heart and breathing have stopped by compressing the chest and forcing air into the lungs.

case log A written record of the cases a person has worked on.

case report A detailed description of what a person did.

domestic animal An animal that is raised by human beings as a pet, work animal, or food source.

ecology The branch of science that studies plants' and animals' relation to each other and the environment.

euthanize To humanely put to death.

inclement Unpleasantly cold, hot, or wet.

inpatient Kept in a medical facility overnight.

intravenous Inserted directly into a vein.

magnetic resonance imaging (MRI) A technology that uses large magnets and electric current to create images of the inside of the body.

neurology The branch of medicine that deals with the nerves, spinal cord, and brain.

oncology The branch of medicine that deals with cancer.

pathology The branch of medicine that deals with the identification of diseases and causes of death.

pharmacology The study of the preparation, application, and effects of medications.

postoperative After surgery.

preoperative Before surgery.

preserve An area where wild animals are protected.

radiology The area of medicine that deals with taking X-rays.

rehabilitation The healing of an injured wild animal to the point where it can be released back into the wild.

synonymous The same as.

traverse To cross.

ultrasound A medical technology that uses sound waves to make images of the inside of a body.

zoology The study of animals.

FOR MORE INFORMATION

American Association of Veterinary State Boards (AAVSB)
380 West 22nd Street, Suite 101
Kansas City, MO 64108
(877) 698-8482 or (816) 931-1504
Website: https://www.aavsb.org
Facebook: @AAVSB
Twitter: @AAVSB
YouTube: https://www.youtube.com/user/aavsbvideos
AAVSB provides state certification and licensing information and tests for veterinary technicians, as well as student services for those studying to be veterinary technicians.

American Society of Animal Science (ASAS)
PO Box 7410
Champaign, IL 61826-7410
(217) 356-9050
Website: https://www.asas.org
Facebook: @American-Society-of-Animal-Science-ASAS
Twitter: @CritterChatter
The ASAS supports research in the field of animal science and provides the latest information on research in the field.

Bureau of Labor Statistics (BLS)
US Department of Labor
Postal Square Building
2 Massachusetts Avenue NE
Washington, DC 20212-0001
(202) 691-5200
Website: https://www.bls.gov
The BLS is the chief federal agency that measures the US

labor market and activity, working conditions, and industry price changes. Each year it researches and compiles information on all types of jobs and employment requirements and updates the *Occupational Outlook Handbook* (https://www.bls.gov/ooh). Thousands of jobs, including those related to veterinary medicine, and their requirements and average salaries are described in the handbook.

Canadian Veterinary Medical Association (CVMA)
339 Booth Street
Ottawa, ON K1R 7K1
Canada
(800) 567-2862 or (613) 236-1162
Website: https://www.canadianveterinarians.net
Facebook: @CanadianVeterinaryMedicalAssociation
Twitter: @https://twitter.com/CanVetMedAssoc
CVMA has a variety of support information for veterinarians and veterinary technicians, including career resources and a journal.

National Association of Veterinary Technicians in American (NAVTA)
PO Box 1227
Albert Lea, MN 56007
(888) 996-2882
Website: https://www.navta.net
Facebook: @VetTechs
Twitter: @VetTechns
NAVTA provides certification for veterinary assistants, veterinary technicians, and specialty veterinary technicians.

Ontario Association of Veterinary Technicians (OAVT)
107–100 Stone Road West
Guelph, ON N1G 5L3
Canada
(800) 675-1859 or (519) 836-4910
Website: http://www.oavt.org
Facebook: @OntarioAssociationOfVeterinaryTechnicians
Twitter: @The_OAVT
OAVT maintains resources for veterinary technicians and
    students, publishes a journal, and includes information
    on volunteer opportunities on its website.

United States Animal Health Association (USAHA)
4221 Mitchell Avenue
Saint Joseph, MO 64507
(816) 671-1144
Website: http://www.usaha.org
Facebook: @USAnimalHealthAssociation
Twitter: @USAnimalHealth
USAHA offers information dealing with the health of
    horses and livestock.

FOR FURTHER READING

Bassert, Joanna M. *McCurnin's Clinical Textbook for Veterinary Technicians*. 9th ed. St. Louis, MO: Elsevier, 2018.

Bedell, J. M. *So, You Want to Work with Animals: Discover Fantastic Ways to Work with Animals, from Veterinary Science to Aquatic Biology*. New York, NY, and Hillsboro, OR: Aladdin and Beyond Words, 2017.

Bjorklund, Ruth. *Wildlife Rescue and Rehabilitation Worker*. New York, NY: Cavendish Square, 2014.

Byers, Ann. *Internship & Volunteer Opportunities for People Who Love Animals*. New York, NY: Rosen Publishing, 2013.

Cambridge Review. *Guide to Veterinary Schools and Careers: Including Profiles on the Top 340 Colleges and Occupational Schools*. San Bernardino, CA: Cambridge Review, 2015.

Campbell, Karen L. *Angell at 100: A Century of Compassionate Care for Animals and Their Families at Angell Animal Medical Center*. Brookline, MA: Lamprey & Lee, 2015.

Christen, Carol, and Richard N. Bolles. *What Color Is Your Parachute? for Teens: Discover Yourself, Design Your Future, and Plan for Your Dream Job*. 3rd ed. New York, NY: Ten Speed Press, 2015.

DeCarlo, Laura. *Resumes for Dummies*. Hoboken, NJ: Wiley, 2015.

Ewing, Susan. *Working with Animals*. Mankato, MN: 12-Story Press, 2018.

Hand, Carol. *Cool Careers Without College for People Who Love Animals*. New York, NY: Rosen Publishing, 2014.

Hemdal, Jay F. *Aquarium Careers.* 3rd rev. ed. CreateSpace Independent Publishing, 2015.

Henke, Scott E., and Paul R. Krausman. *Becoming a Wildlife Professional.* Baltimore, MD: Johns Hopkins University, 2001.

Institute for Career Research. *Careers with Zoos and Aquariums.* Chicago, IL: Institute for Career Research, 2015.

Johnson, Anne. *Veterinary Assistant and Laboratory Animal Caretaker Career: The Insider's Guide to Finding a Job at an Amazing Firm, Acing the Interview & Getting Promoted.* Special ed. CreateSpace Independent Publishing, 2016.

Johnson, Anne. *Veterinary Technologist and Technician Career: The Insider's Guide to Finding a Job at an Amazing Firm, Acing the Interview & Getting Promoted.* CreateSpace Independent Publishing, 2016.

BIBLIOGRAPHY

Academy of Veterinary Dental Technicians. "Credentialing Guidelines." Retrieved February 21, 2018. https://avdt.us/credential-guidelines.

American Association of Equine Veterinary Technicians (AAEVT). "Animal Care Technologies." Retrieved February 21, 2018. http://www.aaevt.org/?page=CertificateProgram.

ASPCA. "Shelter Intake and Surrender: Pet Statistics." Retrieved February 5, 2018. https://www.aspca.org/animal-homelessness/shelter-intake-and-surrender/pet-statistics.

The Balance. "Veterinary Technician Specialties." Retrieved February 21, 2018. https://www.thebalance.com/veterinary-technician-specialties-125817.

Blanchard, Monica, and Jessica Moran. "My On the Job Training Experience as Veterinarian Assistant." Moncton Animal Hospital. April 20, 2017. https://www.monctonanimalhospital.com/job-training-experience-veterinarian-assistant.

IEAS News. "A Day in the Life." September 22, 2013. http://internationalexoticanimalsanctuary.blogspot.ca/2013/09/a-day-in-life.html.

Input Youth. "Animal Care Assistant." Retrieved February 12, 2018. https://www.inputyouth.co.uk/jobguides/job-animalcareassistant.html.

Kramer, Mary Hope. "Animal Health Inspector Career Profile and Salary." August 20, 2017. https://www.thebalance.com/animal-health-inspector-125787?.

Letain, Collin. "My Summer as a Wildlife Technician with the CWHC." CWHC. September 18, 2015. http://blog.healthywildlife.ca/my-summer-as-a-wildlife-technician-with-the-cwhc.

NAVTA. "Veterinary Nurse: The National Credentialing Initiative." October 16, 2017. Retrieved February 12, 2018. http://www.navta.net/?page=VeterinaryNurse.

Norris, Jessica. "A Day in the Life of an Animal Care Assistant." March 5, 2014. http://www.langfordvets .co.uk/news/day-life-animal-care-assistant.

Penn State Dubois. "Wildlife Technology." Retrieved February 19, 2018. http://dubois.psu.edu/wildlife.

Pima Medical Institute. "Veterinary Assistant Program Details." Retrieved February 19, 2018. https://pmi .edu/programs/certificate/veterinary-assistant /learnmore.

Rose, Rebecca, and Carin A. Smith. *Career Choices for Veterinary Technicians: Opportunities for Animal Lovers.* Rev. 1st ed. Lakewood, CO: American Animal Hospital Association Press, 2013.

Royster, Sara. "My Career—Veterinary Technician Lindsay Calhoun." *Occupational Outlook Quarterly*, Spring 2014, pp. 13–14. https://www.bls.gov /careeroutlook/2014/spring/mycareer.pdf.

Rudolph, Heather Wood. "What It's Really Like to Work with Animals at SeaWorld." *Cosmopolitan.* June 28, 2016. http://www.cosmopolitan.com/career/a60655 /seaworld-animal-trainer.

Sokanu.com. "What Does a Veterinary Assistant Do?" Retrieved March 7, 2018. https://www.sokanu.com /careers/veterinary-assistant.

US Bureau of Labor Statistics. *Occupational Outlook Handbook*, Retrieved March 7, 2018. "Animal Care and Service Workers." https://www.bls.gov/ooh /personal-care-and-service/animal-care-and-service -workers.htm. "Environmental Science and Protection."

https://www.bls.gov/ooh/life-physical-and-social
-science/environmental-science-and-protection
-technicians.htm. "Veterinary Assistants and Laboratory
Animal Caretakers. https://www.bls.gov/ooh
/healthcare/veterinary-assistants-and-laboratory-animal
-caretakers.htm. "Veterinary Technologists and
Technicians." https://www.bls.gov/ooh/healthcare
/veterinary-technologists-and-technicians.htm.

VeterinarianEDU.org. "How to Become a Vet Tech."
Retrieved February 19, 2018. https://www
.veterinarianedu.org/vet-tech-careers.

VeterinarianEDU.org. "Steps on How to Become a
Veterinary Assistant in Massachusetts." Retrieved February
19, 2018. https://www.veterinarianedu.org
/massachusetts-veterinary-assistant.

Veterinary Medicine Careers. "All About Large Animal
Practice Veterinary Technicians." Retrieved February 20,
2018. http://veterinarymedicinecareers.org/large
-animal-practice.

Veterinary Medicine Careers. "A Day in the Life of a
Veterinary Care Assistant." Retrieved February 6, 2018.
http://veterinarymedicinecareers
.org/a-day-in-the-life-of-a-veterinary-assistant.

Wilson College. "What's It Like to Be an Equine Veterinary
Medical Technician." Retrieved February 20, 2018.
https://www.wilson.edu/a-day-in-the-life-of-an-equine
-vet-tech.

Worcester Technical High School. "Veterinary Assisting."
Retrieved February 19, 2018. http://techhigh.us
/index.php/veterinary-assisting.

INDEX

H

high school, 7, 16–17, 22–23,
26, 28, 34, 36, 39, 43,
48–49

I

inclement weather, 12
inpatient animals, 16
internal medicine veterinary
technician, 59
internship, 38–40, 43, 45, 48,
49
interview, 41, 47, 49, 53–55,
62
intravenous drip feed, 41

K

kennel attendant, 26

L

language, 38, 49
large animal practice, 6, 12,
18–19, 38, 49, 65
Letain, Collin, 29–30

M

magnetic resonance imaging
(MRI), 21
math, 34–35, 44
mobile veterinary services, 13,
51–52
Moran, Jessica, 4

N

National Association of Veterinary
Technicians in America
(NAVTA), 18–20, 56
networking, 49
neurology, 59

O

oncology, 59
online programs, 22, 34, 43,
44, 46, 64
on-the-job training, 34, 39, 47
outlook, 10

P

pathology, 44, 57
pets, 6, 8, 10, 12–13, 19, 27,
36, 48, 64
pharmacology, 19, 45
postoperative activities, 60
preoperative activities, 41, 60
preserve, 6, 7, 9–10, 15, 26,
27, 30, 65–66

Q

qualities, 24–25

R

radiology, 19
registered veterinary nurse
(RVN), 20
rehabilitation, 15, 23, 38, 62, 66

About the Author

Jeri Freedman has a bachelor's degree from Harvard University. She has more than fifteen years of experience in sales and marketing for high-tech and medical products companies, including the Clinical Assays division of Baxter-Travenol. She enjoys writing career-related books for young adults. Among her published works are *Jump-Starting a Career in Hospitals and Home Health Care*; *Women in the Workplace: Wages, Respect, and Equal Rights*; *Being a Leader: Organizing and Inspiring a Group*; *Careers in Pharmaceutical Sales*; and *Careers in Computer Support*.

Photo Credits